Clinical trial of chloroq

Fatai Adewale Fehintola

Clinical trial of chloroquine-chorpheniramine in malaria

Clinical trial of antimalarial drugs

LAP LAMBERT Academic Publishing

Impressum / Imprint

Bibliografische Information der Deutschen Nationalbibliothek: Die Deutsche Nationalbibliothek verzeichnet diese Publikation in der Deutschen Nationalbibliografie; detaillierte bibliografische Daten sind im Internet über http://dnb.d-nb.de abrufbar. Alle in diesem Buch genannten Marken und Produktnamen unterliegen warenzeichen-, marken- oder patentrechtlichem Schutz bzw. sind Warenzeichen oder eingetragene Warenzeichen der jeweiligen Inhaber. Die Wiedergabe von Marken, Produktnamen, Gebrauchsnamen, Handelsnamen, Warenbezeichnungen u.s.w. in diesem Werk berechtigt auch ohne besondere Kennzeichnung nicht zu der Annahme, dass solche Namen im Sinne der Warenzeichen- und Markenschutzgesetzgebung als frei zu betrachten wären und daher von jedermann benutzt werden dürften.

Bibliographic information published by the Deutsche Nationalbibliothek: The Deutsche Nationalbibliothek lists this publication in the Deutsche Nationalbibliografie; detailed bibliographic data are available in the Internet at http://dnb.d-nb.de. Any brand names and product names mentioned in this book are subject to trademark, brand or patent protection and are trademarks or registered trademarks of their respective holders. The use of brand names, product names, common names, trade names, product descriptions etc. even without a particular marking in this works is in no way to be construed to mean that such names may be regarded as unrestricted in respect of trademark and brand protection legislation and could thus be used by anyone.

Coverbild / Cover image: www.ingimage.com

Verlag / Publisher:
LAP LAMBERT Academic Publishing
ist ein Imprint der / is a trademark of
AV Akademikerverlag GmbH & Co. KG
Heinrich-Böcking-Str. 6-8, 66121 Saarbrücken, Deutschland / Germany
Email: info@lap-publishing.com

Herstellung: siehe letzte Seite /
Printed at: see last page
ISBN: 978-3-659-41555-5

Zugl. / Approved by: Nigeria,National Postgraduate Medical College, Diss.,1999

DEDICATION

For me, I have set my face,
Firmly and truly towards Him
Who created the heavens and the earth
And never shall I give partners to God.

To: **Remi,**

      Moji,

            Omotayo

CONTENTS

Chapter 1: INTRODUCTION

Chapter 2: MATERIALS AND METHODS

ACKNOWLEDGEMENTS

I am greatly indebted to my friend (as he is wont to call me) and supervisor, Professor Akintude Sowunmi, for his moral and financial support. I sincerely thank Prof. A.M.J. Oduola for his contribution towards completion of this project.

Mr. Akande, Miss Owoyokun and Mrs. Fatima Fawunmi did well by typing this work; Miss Joke Ishola, my able assistant, deserves special mention for her immense efforts at the clinic. Prof. Falase, Drs. Ogunbiyi and Salako, and Mr. Akangbe helped in overcoming the initial inertia. Mr Olomu and Mr. Fajimi provided laboratory back-up, I thank them all. Dr. A.A. Adeyemo assisted me with the analysis of the data. I am grateful to him.

I express my sincere gratitude to my wife (Adelayo) for her unflinching support and Abdul Basit for his patience. Above all is my Lord God, ALMIGHTY ALLAH, THE BENEFICENT who taught by the pen, who provided me with the numerous human and material resources to be able to start and complete this programme in spite of all odds.

This study received financial support from UNDP/World Bank/WHO Special Programme for Research and Training in Tropical Diseases.

LIST OF TABLES

5

INTRODUCTION

Introduction

Malaria is a protozoan disease transmitted by the bite of female anopheles mosquitoes. It is a major cause of morbidity and mortality in the endemic areas of the world. An estimated 40% of the world population is at risk of infection and about 300 - 500 million people are said to infected worldwide[1]. In 1989, about 52 million cases were reported globally excluding Africa. Thirty-nine percent of these were recorded in India, 11% in Brazil and another 25% originated from Thailand, Sri Lanka, Afghanistan, Viet-Nam, China, and Myanmar. Malaria incidence in America increased from 27000 cases in 1974 to 1.1 million in 1979, 52% of which came from Brazil[1].

In sub-Saharan Africa, the morbidity and mortality from malaria is high, with about 1 million children dying of the disease annually[2]. Majority of deaths occur in children below the age of 5 years in the order: 6 per 1000 (10%) in 0-1 year old, 11 per 1000 (24%) in children 1-4 years old. The disease is one of the leading causes of childhood mortality in Nigeria; it is responsible for an estimated 300,000 deaths every year[3].

Four species of Plasmodium infect man. These are *Plasmodium falciparum, Plasmodium vivax, Plasmodium ovale and Plasmodium malariae. P. falciparum* is the most lethal of all the human species and it accounts for most of the infections in Africa and for over a third of the infections in the rest of the world[4].

In Nigeria, *P. falciparum* is responsible for 85-90% of all malaria infections[5]. *P. vivax* is hardly encountered. Cerebral malaria is the most dreaded complication of *P. falciparum*. Other notable acute complications include anaemia with or without cardiac failure, renal impairment, metabolic derangement, abortion, intra-uterine growth retardation, and pulmonary oedema amongst others.

Life cycle of Plasmodium

The life cycle of genus Plasmodium consists of complex asexual reproductive phases in man and both sexual and asexual phases in female Anopheles mosquito. The biphasic asexual cycle in man begins with sporozoites inocculation when an infective mosquito attempts to take a blood meal. The sporozoites as soon as released into capillarries and venules disappear into the liver within 30-60 minutes to begin pre-erythrocytic schizogony. The sprorozoites develop within the hepatocytes to form hepatic trophozoites and schizont with eventual rupture of the hepatocytes to release merozoites. This development within the liver usually lasts 5-7 days for *P. falciparum* and up to 15 days for *P. malariae* while *P. vivax and P. ovale*, the Plasmodium species responsible for malaria relapse require 8-9 days. A proportion of the sporozoites of *P. vivax and P. ovale* do not divide immediately, remaining dormant for months before reproduction begins. Malaria relapses have been ascribed to these hypnozoites[6 &7].

The merozoites released from the hepatocytes invade the red blood cells to begin the second phase of asexual cycle in man. Invasion of erythrocytes requires a specific surface receptor. In *P. vivax* this is related to Duffy blood group antigen (fy^a of fy^b) which is lacking in most West Africans. People of this region are therefore resistant to infection by this Plasmodium species. During invasion, the merozoite first orientates so that its apical end is attached to the erythrocyte surface and then interiorizes itself so as to lie within an intra-erythrocytic parasitophorous vacuole. During the early stage of development the "young rings" (immature trophozoites) of the four species appear similar under light microscopy. As the trophozoites enlarge, species-specific characteristics become evident, pigment becomes visible, and the parasite assumes an irregular or amoeboid shape. Erythrocytic cycle usually lasts 48 h except in *P. malariae* when it takes 72 h to complete. The immature trophozoites feed on host's haemoglobin to develop to mature trophoizoites then undergo nuclear fission (schizogony)

8

and, eventual release of 6-8 merozoites in *P. falciparum* and 16-24 in the others. The resultant merozoites are capable of invading red cells and repeating the cycle. After a series of such asexual cycles some of the parasites develop into morphologically distinct sexual forms (gametocytes) which are long lived and incapable of further development in man.

Life cycle in female anopheles mosquito begins with the fusion of male and female gametocytes in the midgut following their ingestion with blood meal. This so called extrinsic cycle usually lasts at least 7 days depending on the ambient temperature. The result of the fusion of micro (male) and macro-(female) gametocytes is a motile zygote called ookinete. The second phase of development in the mosquito is asexual reproduction. It commences with penetration of gut wall of the mosquito by the ookinete and subsequent encystment to form oocyst. The resulting oocyst expands by asexual division until it bursts to liberate myriad of sporozoites which then migrate to the salivary gland to await inoculation into another human at the next feeding.

The success of Plasmodium species as a parasite of man (and other primates) hinges on certain survival mechanisms. Some of these include an almost instantaneous disappearance into the hepatocytes of sporozoite following inoculation by the mosquito. This has been adduced as part of the reasons for partial rather than complete immunity that occurs in endemic areas[8]. Pre-erythrocytic development in the hepatocytes also results in multiplication of each sporozoite thus 30,000 merozoites are released per infected hepatocytes in *P. falciparum* infection and 10-15,000 in the others. Also, *P. vivax* and *P. ovale* both have hypnozoites which are not only sources of erythrocytes infective merozoites but potential gametocyte and sporozoites in manifold. Further, *P. falciparum* singularly exhibits notoriety of cyto-adherence in the infected erythrocytes. Development of cerebral malaria and some other life threatening complications of falciparum malaria have been attributed to this phenomenon. Lack of expression of major histocompatibility antigen (MHC) by erythrocytes and therefore lack of recognition by T cells is also a survival mechanism by this organism. Additional multiplication is also seen when each infecting merozoite from the liver undergoes schizogony (erythrocytic) to produce between 6 and 24 daughter merozoites. And in the mosquito each pair (micro- and macro-gametocytes) produces thousands of sprozoites to ensure continued survival. Even when acquired through unnatural means, for example, blood transfusion, the Plasmodium merozoites have enough provision to establish erythrocytic shizogony, eventual sporogony and continued survival.

Figure 1 showing the illustrated life cycle of malaria parasite

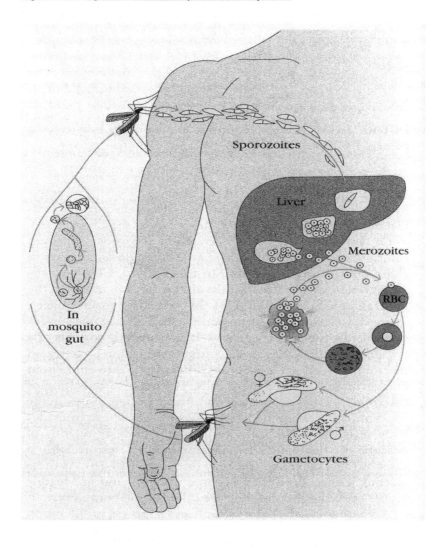

Clinical Presentation of falciparum malaria

In general, the presenting symptoms in malaria follow rupture of parasitized erythrocytes with the release of cytokines. Classically, the symptoms of fever and chills occur every 48 or 72 hours. Myalgia, arthralgia, headache, malaise, nausea and vomiting and anorexia may also be present. Children under the age of five years may have febrile convulsion. Other forms of presentation as a result of complications may be seen, thus coma as a result of cerebral malaria, jaundice, anaemia and anaemic heart failure are all possible in severe malaria.

Unusual presentation in acute uncomplicated malaria may include such clinical features as psychosis[9], mononeuritis multiplex[10], pruritus, epigastric pain with or without vomiting or diarrhoea, cough and chest pain. It is pertinent to note that malaria could be the only explanation for some of these presentations and any of these may be the only feature seen in certain groups of patients for example, a child's only complaint may be epigastic pain and subsequent confirmation and treatment for malaria cures the illness (Sowunmi A., personal communication)

Diagnosis of malaria

Presumptive diagnosis of malaria is clinical though, appropriate laboratory confirmation is desirable where facilities are available. On occasions when malaria presents with certain uncommon clinical features the task of diagnosis becomes daunting if not impossible. Laboratory confirmation of malaria rests on the demonstration of asexual forms of the parasite in the peripheral blood smears stained with one of the Romanowsky stains (Giemsa; Wright; Field, or Leishman's at p H 7.2). Both thick and thin smears should be examined under oil immersion. The thin smear must be air dried and fixed with methanol. The parasitemia is expressed as the number of parasitized erythrocytes in 1000 cells and then converted to the number per micro-litre. In the case of thick smear, staining is done without fixing. And as many layers of erythrocytes overlie each other and, are then lysed during the staining procedure, the thick film has the advantage of concentrating the parasites, and therefore increasing the sensitivity of diagnosis. Both parasites and white cells are counted and the number of parasites per microliter calculated from leukocyte count. A minimum of 200 white cells should be counted.

So far, microscopy remains the gold standard for qualitative and quantitative assessment of parasite load. The sensitivity is not 100% and occasionally, asexual forms may be missed in the thin film and, interpretation of thick smear may require experienced microscopist to avoid misdiagnosis.

Other laboratory diagnostic techniques include (i) Quantitative buffy coat (QBC)[11] which requires far more financial resources and is less sensitive than microscopy; (ii) determination of parasite-specific lactate dehydrogenase (pLDH)[12] (iii) detection of parasite deoxyribonucleic acid (PCR amplified DNA detection by gel electrophoresis) and, (iv) parasite specific antigen detection (parasight- F test), which has been found to compare favourably with microscopy in terms of sensitivity, specificity and positive predictive value[13] [14]. Being available as a dipstick it requires little expertise. However, parasite quantification is less than perfect.

Present status of falciparum malaria therapy

In view of the enormous cost, operational and technical problems encountered by malaria eradication programme, emphasis on malaria control has now shifted to reducing morbidity and mortality through prompt diagnosis and adequate treatment.

From the early 1950s until recently, chloroquine given at the recommended dose of 25 mg per kilogramme of body weight over three days was the mainstay of therapy because of its high efficacy and safety, ready availability, and low cost. Recent reports, however, indicate significant decline in the sensitivity of *Plasmodium falciparum* to chloroquine with treatment failures as high as 50% in some parts of Nigeria[15]. In East Africa and Southeast Asia sensitivity to this drug is very low. The first cases of chloroquine-resistant malaria were from South America and Southeast Asia in 1959 and 1960, respectively[16]. It has since become a

13

global phenomenon. In 1978, resistance to chloroquine was demonstrated in *P. falciparum* from East Africa beginning in Kenya and the United Republic of Tanzania[17] [18]. In Nigeria, *Plasmodium falciparum* showing reduced sensitivity to chloroquine was documented in the last decade[19].

Amodiaquine, given at a dose of 25-30 mg per kg orally over 3 day period, has been employed in the treatment of acute uncomplicated falciparum malaria. Although marginally effective in the treatment of chloroquine resistant malaria, resistance to this 4-hydroxyanilin-substituted quinoline compound largely follows the distribution of chloroquine resistance. It is also more likely to cause hepatic damage and bone marrow depression[20] [21]. Therefore, its frequent use in endemic areas should, at the moment, be actively discouraged until more is known about its toxicity in children from endemic areas[22].

Pyrimethamine-sulphadoxine (P-S) containing 25 mg of pyrimethmine and 500mg sulphadoxine is another drug commonly used in areas of chloroquine resistant *Plasmodium falciparum*[23]. The drug is given as a single dose of 3 tablets for adults. In children, P-S is administered according to body weight. A single dose of half tablet is given to children 5-10 kg body weight, 1 tablet to dose 11-20 kg, and one and half to dose 21-30 kg. High sensitivity of falciparum malaria to P-S has been demonstrated in some studies in Nigeria[24, 25]. However, P-S is slow to act and is not recommended for severe malaria despite the availability of parenteral formulation. Its adverse effects include allergic skin reactions, abdominal pain with diarrhoea[26]. Also considerable resistance has been reported in Southeast Asia and East Africa as well as in some parts of Nigeria[27] [28].

Mefloquine is a quinoline-methanol which can be used in both acute uncomplicated and chemoprophylaxis of malaria. It is effective in both sensitive and multidrug resistant strains of falciparum malaria. It is available in oral formulation only. The usual dosage is 15-25 mg per kg body weight given as a single dose or in two divided doses at 6 hours interval. It has a very long half life. Mefloquine is the first-line drug of choice in areas of multidrug resistant malaria like Thailand. The drug may cause abdominal pain and vomiting which might result

14

in low drug concentrations thus leading to treatment failure[29]. Psychosis may also occur during treatment with mefloquine[30] Oduola *et al*, reported primary *in vitro* resistance of P. falciparum to mefloquine in Nigeria[31]. Recent *in vivo* studies however, revealed full sensitivity to this drug[28]

Halofantrine is a 9-phenanthrene methanol schizonticidal antimalaria drug. It has been shown to be effective in treatment of multi-drug resistant strains of *P. falciparum[32]*. The recommended dose for adult is 500 mg every 6 h for three doses and for children it is given at a dose of 8 mg per kg body weight[33]. Halofantrine is poorly absorbed and has a low bioavailability which is often increased by fatty foods[34]. This poses a great problem since malaria patients are likely to be in fasting state during drug administration. This low bioavailability coupled with its short half-life of 2-3 hours may lead to the development of resistance to halofantrine, because low drug concentrations may enable the parasites to withstand treatment. Resistance to halofantrine is also on the increase for example, response of *P. falciparum* at introduction into Nigeria in early 1990s was 95-100%[35]. Recent reports from both eastern and western parts of Nigeria revealed sensitivity of 89-90.5%[27].

The history of the use of quinine in the treatment of malaria dates back to around 1630 in Peru. The drug is effective in the treatment of acute uncomplicated and complicated falciparum malaria. However, in Southeast Asia, increasing quinine tolerance is encountered[36, 37] and combinations of quinine with antibiotics like tetracycline, erythromycin have been found effective[38]. It is available in tablets and injectable forms. The latter is employed in severe and complicated malaria. The earliest record of antimalarial drug resistance was that of *P. falciparum* to quinine reported from Brazil in 1910[39, 40]. In Nigeria, *P. falciparum* is fully sensitive to quinine[22] and, quinine is the recommended initial treatment for severe and complicated malaria.

The artemisinin group of drugs is derived from *artemisia annua L,* a chinese herbal treatment for fevers[41]. Artemether, artesunate and other drugs in this group contain the sesquiterpene lactone ring and are rapidly schizonticidal. Artemether now compares favourably well with

15

quinine in the treatment of cerebral malaria[42, 43]. The artemisinin derivatives are effective in multidrug resistant strains of *P. falciparum*[44-47]. They are also devoid of serious side effects even during pregnancy[48].

Drug therapy in severe and complicated malaria in areas of chloroquine-sensitive falciparum malaria may include chloroquine given as 5 mg per kg body weight into 5% dextrose or normal saline over 2-4 h at 12 hourly to a total dose of 25 mg/kg body weight. Quinine with or without a loading dose given as intravenous infusion in normal saline or 5% dextrose over 4 hours at 8 hourly interval remains the treatment of choice in severe and complicated malaria. Artemether has also been used in treatment of cerebral malaria with comparable outcome to quinine and chloroquine treatment[49]. The usual regimen is 3.2 mg per kg body weight as a loading dose followed by 1.6 mg per kg body weight given daily for 4 days.

Combination chemotherapy for *P. falciparum* malaria

The aim of combination chemotherapy is to enhance efficacy of the combined drugs and to retard development of resistance. Ideally the combined drugs should have similar pharmacokinetics and pharmacodynamics and should display no enhanced adverse effects. The combination of quinine and tetracycline has been widely used in Southeast Asia, and quinine plus sulphadoxine-pyrimethamine more frequently in South America[50]. In contrast to tetracyclines, clindamycin can be used in children and combinations of clindamycin with quinine or chloroquine seem to be more effective than combinations with quinine-tetracyclines or chloroquine-doxycycline[50]. The major disadvantage of quinine alone or in combination with antibiotics is the long duration of therapy. Recently combinations of mefloquine-pyrimathimine-sulphadoxine (MPS) and, atovaquone plus proguanil were introduced. In Thailand, as well as in Nigeria, MPS was not therapeutically superior to mefloquine alone[28]. In contrast, the MPS combination has been highly effective in some parts of Africa even in reduced recommended dosage[50]. The atovaquone-proguanil combination has not only been successful in treating acute infections, it is being considered as a chemo-prophylactic agent. Trial to evaluate the tolerability and efficacy for this purpose

16

is underway in Kenya and Gabon[50]. Other suggested combinations include artemether-mefloquine[51], artemether plus sulphadoxine-pyrimethamine. Many of these combinations require optimisation of dosage, timing and application.

The combination of antimalarial drugs with non-antimalarial drugs followed reports of successful *in vitro* reversal of chloroquine resistance with verapamil[52.] This subject is dealt with in more details later in this dissertation.

Mechanism of chloroquine resistant malaria

Drug resistance can be defined as the ability of a cell or an organism to survive in the presence of higher concentration of a given drug than would originally have been expected. The global resurgence of malaria is due mainly to the advent of drug resistant parasites and insecticide resistant mosquito vectors[53, 54].

The mechanism of resistance of *P falciparum* to chloroquine remains to be fully elucidated. There is, however, conclusive evidence that resistant strains of *P. falciparum* accumulate far less chloroquine than the sensitive strains[55]. The drug target that is responsible for chloroquine action in *P. falciparum* is not known, however, it has been shown that vacuolar concentrations of chloroquine necessary to inhibit parasite growth increase with drug resistance, indicating a reduction in the susceptibility of a plausible target to the drug. Slower rate of proton pumping into the vacuole with consequent truncation of pH drive for acidotropic drug accumulation has, therefore, been considered as a veritable explanation for chloroquine resistance. It has also been considered that resistant strains of *P. falciparum* may have a mechanism that ensures continuous proton leak from its vacuole thus reducing acidotropic drug accumulation to toxic level. Factors that may be responsible for this down regulation remain poorly elucidated. The suggestion that *P. falciparum* chloroquine resistant strains express a multidrug resistant gene (Pfmdr 1 and Pfmdr 2) similar to that found in chemotherapy resistant cancer cells also remains largely inconclusive[56].

17

Reversal of antimalaria drug resistance in *P. falciparum*

The discovery of an isolate of *P. falciparum* (from Thailand) that showed multiple resistances to mefloquine, chloroquine and quinine stimulated interest in the possible similarity (ies) between multi-drug resistant cancer cells and multidrug resistant *Plasmodium falciparum*. Since 1987 when verapamil, a calcium channel blocker, was successfully used to reverse resistance to chloroquine in *P. falciparum*, several other agents have been tried and these include:-chlorpromazine, desipramine and antihistamines[57] [58] [59]. So far reversal of resistance in *P. falciparum* has been achieved for chloroquine, mefloquine, quinine and quinidine[60] [61] [62].

The mechanism of resistant reversing drugs in falciparum malaria remains largely undetermined. However, multidrug-resistant cancer cells prevent accumulation of drugs to toxic level by active efflux of the drugs. If this active efflux is inhibited, the drug then accumulates and the resistant cells again become sensitive. Verapamil inhibits this active efflux. The exact mechanism by which verapamil inhibits efflux of anticancer drugs from resistant cancer cells is yet to be fully elucidated. This has been ascribed to the ability of verapamil to bind to 150 - 170 kilodalton membrane-associated glycoproteins which appears to bind cytotoxic drugs at an allosteric site with consequent efflux from the multidrug resistant cells. The currently known resistant reversing drugs in drug resistant *P. falciparum* might have a similar mechanism to what is found in resistant cancer cells.

It has been hypothesized that chloroquine-resistance in *P. falciparum* is due to a similar failure of the drug to reach toxic levels within the parasite because of an acquired enhanced active efflux of this drug. If the foregoing were true, it is also expected that verapamil and other agents used in reversing resistance in cancer cells would have similar effects in resistant malaria parasite. Further, resistant reversing agents will not affect the 50% inhibitory concentration (IC_{50}) of chloroquine against the sensitive strains of *P. falciparum*. Indeed, *in vitro* studies have so far shown that resistant reversing drugs are able to reduce 50% inhibitory concentrations of resistant *P. falciparum* but had no such effect on sensitive strains[63]. Recent reports indicate that resistance reversal can be demonstrated *in vitro* and *in vivo* in *P. falciparum* resistant to chloroquine[63].

18

Because this dissertation is focused on three drugs chloroquine, chlorpheniramine and halofantrine, the pharmacological properties of these drugs are briefly described below.

Chloroquine

Chloroquine (7-chloro-4-(4-diethylamino-1-methyl butyl amino-quinoline), Figure 1, is a chemotherapeutic agent for the clinical treatment of malaria. Chloroquine was first synthesized in 1934 by German chemists. It was then considered too toxic despite proven antimalarial effect. Rediscovery and further evaluation in 1941, however, revealed no serious toxicity.

Chloroquine is available in oral, rectal and as intramuscular and intravenous formulations. It is water soluble and rapidly absorbed following oral or parenteral administration in adults with malaria of moderate severity. Its bioavailability following oral medication is 70%. In children with uncomplicated malaria given an initial treatment dose of 10 mg base/kg as tablets, peak plasma concentrations of approximately 250 ug/ liter were reached in 2 hours. Intramuscular and subcutaneous administrations of chloroquine give almost identical plasma or whole blood concentration profiles. Preliminary studies with chloroquine suppositories suggest rectal bioavailability less than half of oral but sustained therapeutic blood concentration may be achieved[64].

The total apparent volume of distribution is enormous because of extensive tissue binding. The profile of blood concentration after parenteral administration is characterized by sharp peak with wide peak to trough variation. For intramuscular and subcutaneous administration small frequent doses (e.g. 3.5 mg base/kg 6 hourly or 2.5 mg 4 hourly are preferred as it avoids toxic peak concentrations. Chloroquine concentrations in red cells are approximately three times higher than in plasma and there is considerable concentration in granulocytes and platelets. Whole blood concentrations are 6-10 times higher than plasma concentrations. Chloroquine is 55% protein-bound in plasma; concentrations in the cerebrospinal fluid are very low with a mean value of 2.7% of corresponding whole blood concentrations.

19

Chloroquine is 51% cleared unchanged by the kidney the remainder is biotransformed by the liver, mainly to desethyl- and bisdesethyl chloroquine. Elimination is reduced in renal failure but this is irrelevant in acute malaria, that is, dosage need not be reduced[65]. The principal metabolite desethyl chloroquine has similar activity with that of chloroquine against sensitive *P. falciparum* but in resistant strains desethyl-chloroquine has significantly less activity than chloroquine[66]. For curative treatment (therapeutic blood concentration) the half life of chloroquine is about 6-10 days.

Oral chloroquine is usually well tolerated. Acute toxic effects like nausea, headache, uneasiness and dysphoria are relatively common but seldom serious. Patients may vomit and may complain of blurred vision. Postural hypotension associated with malaria may be worsened and pruritus can sometimes be severe. Pruritus may respond to steroids but not to antihitamines[67]. Parenteral chloroquine is a potent vasodilator. There are several reports of sudden death following administration of intramuscular chloroquine to children with severe malaria[68, 69]. These deaths probably result from cardiovascular toxicity. Chloroquine overdose may manifest with coma, convulsion, dysarrhythmias and hypotension. Diazepam is a specific antidote[70]. Acute neuropsychiatric (psychosis, dyskinesia, tremor, hearing loss) reactions to chloroquine may occur.

Retina damage remains the most feared complication of chronic chloroquine usage. Significant risk of retinopathy is associated with administration of more than 100 g of chloroquine to adult. Skeletal or cardiac myopathy may occur in patients receiving high maintenance dose therapy for rheumatoid arthritis[71].

Chlorpheniramine

Chlorpheniramine maleate, chlorprophen-1-pyridamine maleate, Figure 2, is a potent, highly effective and widely used antihistaminic drug[72]. Its use in the treatment of allergic rhinitis started in the early 1950s. Other important indications for chlorpheniramine include pruritus, anaphylaxis, urticaria and hay fever. In Nigeria, and in other countries in Africa chlorpheniramine has been employed in the treatment or prevention of chloroquine induced pruritus.

Chlorpheniramine is available in oral and parenteral formulations. The drug is well absorbed after oral administration, peak concentration appearing within 2-3 hours. The recommended oral adult dose is 12-24 mg in divided doses or 0.4 mg/kg body weight in (3 daily) divided doses in children.

Following oral administration, a half life of 12-15 hours has been reported though, plasma level after four hours is sub-therapeutic requiring repeated administration[73]. The drug is extensively distributed throughout the body with an apparent volume of distribution of about 255% of the body weight. It is about 70% bound to plasma protein and undergoes enterohepatic circulation[72].

Chlorpheniramine is extensively metabolised to form polar and non-polar metabolites. Studies have indicated two metabolites, mono- and di-demethylchlorpheniramine result from N-alkylation of the drug[72]. It is excreted in the urine both as the parent drug as well as metabolites. About 1% is also excreted via the faeces.

Drowsiness is a well known side effect of most of the older antihistamines including chlorpheniramine. Other side effects include headache, psychomotor impairment, antimuscarinic effects such as urinary retention, dry mouth, blurred vision and gastrointestinal disturbances, occasional rashes and photosensitivity reactions have also been reported; paradoxical stimulation may rarely occur, especially in high dosage or in children[74].

Halofantrine

Halofantrine, a phenanthrene-methanol, is a product of the antimalarial drug programme of the Walter Reed Army Institute of Research (Washington, DC, USA). It is an effective alternative in drug sensitive and drug resistant falciparum malaria. There is no parenteral formulation for general use thus its application is mainly in acute uncomplicated malaria.

Halofantrine, Figure 3, is 3-(dibutylamino)-1-(1, 3-dichloro-6-(trifluoromethyl)-9-phenanthryl) propan-1-ol. The currently available formulation, halofantrine hydrochloride, is poorly and erratically absorbed from gastrointestinal tract as a result of its limited solubility. Ingestion of food, especially fatty meal significantly increases its absorption. However, the micronized preparation, still undergoing evaluation, has shown better bioavailability[75].

The estimated apparent volume of distribution is large. Halofantrine is almost entirely eliminated by hepatic biotransformation. The estimated terminal half life is 3-4 days. The principal metabolite, desbutyl-halofantrine has equal biological activity but is cleared more slowly than the parent compound. Halofantrine concentrates more in plasma than red blood cells. It undergoes enterohepatic circulation. Excretion is via the kidneys either as the halofantrine or the desbutyl-metabolite.

The drug is generally well tolerated in children. Abdominal pain and diarrhoea are the most commonly encountered side-effects but they are usually mild and self limited. Pruritus has been reported in 13% of Nigerians[26]. Sudden death and bizarre cardiac arrhythmias have been reported in adults taking halofantrine in the usual recommended dose of 24 mg/Kg in three divided doses over 12 hours[76, 77].

23

Previous studies on the combination of chloroquine and antihistamines for reversal of chloroquine resistance in *P. falciparum*

In vitro studies:

Following the report of chloroquine resistance reversing effect of verapamil[52], further efforts were directed toward obtaining effective but less toxic alternatives. Peters, *et al,* [59] demonstrated resistance reversing effect of tricyclic antihistaminic in *P. falciparum in vitro* and in Aotus monkeys. Basco *et al*,[58] assessed resistance reversing effects of cyproheptadine, azatidine and loratidine in culture adapted strains of *P. falciparum*. In the latter (study) activity enhancement index (AEI) was calculated for various concentrations of chloroquine and antihistaminics to determine potentiating effect or otherwise of the antihistamine employed. The study demonstrated resistance reversing effect(s) of cyproheptidine and azatidine while loratidine was completely devoid of chloroquine-potentiating action. It remains to be determined, however, the exact mechanism(s) of reversal in any of the agents so far employed. Whatever the mechanism(s) involved available evidence suggests that reversal may be dose-dependent[58].

In vivo studies

There are limited clinical studies on the combination of chloroquine and potential resistance reversing compounds. Addition of desipramine to chloroquine in the treatment of chloroquine resistant falciparum malaria showed no therapeutic advantage over chloroquine alone[78]. This apparent lack of effect may be attributable to the high plasma protein binding of desipramine[79]. In more recent trials, the addition of chlorpheniramine to chloroquine apparently produced clinical reversal in patients with chloroquine resistant malaria[63] and this reversal correlated closely with reversal *in vitro*. The latter study, a double blind placebo controlled study compared chloroquine plus placebo with chloroquine plus chlorpheniramine in acute uncomplicated falciparum malaria in children. The study showed 85% cure rate for the chloroquine-chlorpheniramine and a cure of 75% of those treated with chloroquine plus placebo. Although no statistical significance was demonstrated in the cure rate between the

24

two treatment regimens, some of the patients successfully treated with chloroquine-chlorpheniramine demonstrated *in vitro* resistance to chloroquine.

The combination of chloroquine with chlorpheniramine has also demonstrated better efficacy when compared with sulphadoxine-pyrimethamine[80]. Although, doses of chlorpheniramine used in the two clinical trials were relatively high, the latter more than the former, no serious adverse effect was reported. Promethazine, another antihistamine, is more potent than chlorpheniramine at reversing resistance in *P. falciparum in vitro* (Sowunmi, personal communication). However, because promethazine produces more sedation, it has not been favoured for clinical trials in children (Sowunmi, personal communication).

Background to the present study

Chloroquine resistance is increasing in Nigeria[15, 63] and elsewhere. This has posed a serious obstacle to continuing therapeutic effectiveness of chloroquine. The discovery that resistance in *P. falciparum* can be modulated by certain non-antimalarial drugs raises hope for prolonging the clinical use of chloroquine. Recent studies indicate that the combination of chloroquine with chlorpheniramine is superior to chloroquine alone and to pyrimethamine-sulphadoxine in the treatment of falciparum malaria. However, comparison with antimalarial drugs effective in chloroquine resistant malaria, for example halofantrine, and the efficacy and safety of the combination of chloroquine plus chlorpheniramine in children, a group most at risk for malaria, have not been evaluated. It is for these reasons that the study reported in dissertation was planned.

Aims of the present study

The aims of the present studies are

1. To determine the clinical efficacy of the combination of chloroquine plus chlorpheniramine in children suffering from acute symptomatic uncomplicated falciparum malaria.

2. To assess, on a limited basis, the safety of the combination of chloroquine plus chlorpheniramine in the treatment of acute uncomplicated falciparum malaria.

3. To compare the efficacy and safety of chloroquine-chlorpheniramine with halofantrine, a drug effective in the treatment of uncomplicated chloroquine-resistant falciparum malaria in our area of study.

Chapter 2

Materials and Methods

Location

The study was carried out at the Clinical Pharmacology Department of the University College Hospital Ibadan, Nigeria. The patients were drawn from those reporting at the general out-patient department of the hospital.

Patients

A total of 105 children were enrolled into the study (see Appendix 1 for sample size calculation).

Inclusion criteria:

Patients were included into the study if the following criteria were satisfied:

-Age 6 months to 14 years.

-Fever or history of fever in the 24-48 h preceeding presentation.

-Pure *P. falciparum* parasitaemia with a parasite density of at least 1000 asexual forms per microlitre of blood.

-Symptoms compatible with acute uncomplicated falciparum malaria.

-Negative urine test for antimalarial e.g Dill-Glazko(4-aminoquinolines) and lignin - (sulphonamide) (see Appendices 2 & 3).

-Written informed consent

-No concomitant illness, for example bronchopneumonia.

Exclusion criteria:

Patients were excluded from the study if:

-There was severe and complicated malaria.

-There was sickle cell anaemia.

27

-Lignin and/ or Dill-Glazko tests were positive.

-Consent was not given

Withdrawal criteria:

A patient was withdrawn from the study if:

-There was failure to retain oral medication

-There was violation of protocol, for example, failure to attend follow-up clinic

-It was the parent's or guardian's wish to withdraw the child from the study.

-The child developed concomitant illness

-The child developed severe or complicated malaria, for example, cerebral malaria during the study

Conduct of study

Each child underwent physical examination before enrolment into the study. Thereafter weight and axillary temperature were taken and recorded in a form designed for that purpose. Thick and thin blood smears were obtained in an aseptic manner. These were then stained and examined for parasite type and quantification. Thereafter, the children were randomly allotted to either of the two treatment regimens.

Drug treatment and follow up

A child received either of the following treatment:

1 Chloroquine base 30 mg/kg body weight orally over 3 days, that is, 10 mg daily for 3 consecutive days, plus chlorpheniramine 6 mg at enrolment followed by 4 mg 8 hourly if the child was aged 5 years and below, or 8 mg at enrolment followed by 6 mg 8 hourly for 7 days if the child was over 5 years of age (This dosing regimen was modified from a previous study of the efficacy of chloroquine- chlorpheniramine combination in acute falciparum in children[63 80].

2 Halofantrine 8 mg/kg body weight orally 6 hourly for 3 doses.

Chloroquine and chlorpheniramine tablets obtained from the University College Hospital pharmacy were used. These were crushed before mixing with some water in a clean cup and then carefully poured on the tongue in the very young children. The relatively older children were persuaded to swallow the tablets under direct supervision.

In all, the 3 doses of chloroquine and one of the 3 daily doses of chlorpheniramine were directly administered by me. The other 2 doses of chlorpheniramine were given to the parents/guardians to be administered at home at specified times. The parents or guardians were interviewed in respect of drug administration at home.

Halofantrine was obtained directly from the *Smithkline-Beecham, Lagos* in tablet and syrup forms. The very young children were given syrup while the older children received the medication in tablet form. The required dose of the syrup was measured with syringe into clean cup for the children to swallow; the cup was thereafter rinsed with some water to complete each medication. Two doses of halofantrine were administered while the patients were in the clinic and third dose carefully measured into a clean bottle with a clear instruction for its administation at home.

Each child was kept under observation for 6-8 hours to ensure that drugs were not vomited, and to provide opportunity for second dose in the halofantrine group. The children were seen daily for 8 days (days 0-7) and on day 14. At enrolment and on day 7, 2.5 ml of blood each was collected for blood biochemistry and complete blood count. Haemoglobin genotype and glucose 6-phosphate dehydrogenase (G6PD) were determined on day 0. At each daily visit, parents or guardians were asked to describe how "take-home" drugs were administered to ascertain proper medication. The parents/guardians were also questioned on how the children felt with particular reference to resolution or worsening of presenting symptoms and/or appearance of new symptoms whilst on drugs. Further, direct questions, were asked about commonly encountered side effects of the drugs of study. Physical examination including-temperature, pulse, respiration was performed daily before thick smears were done for parasite quantification. Folic acid tablet (5 mg) was given to all children daily for 14 days of the follow up. Paracetamol at a dose of 10-15 mg/kg body weight was given for 24-36 h at 8 hourly intervals for symptomatic relief of fever. Children with temperature above 39°C were also exposed to fan and tepid sponged to bring down the body temperature.

Staining of Blood films for Malaria parasite identification and quantification

Thick and thin films were prepared by pricking the patient on the finger having cleansed with methylated spirit. The third finger was most commonly used while avoiding the thumb. A single drop was collected on a slide for the thin film and two or three drops for the thick film. A spreader was used in completing the preparation of the thin film before fixing with methanol. Thick films were air-dried before staining with 20% Giemsa stain[81].

Giemsa stained blood films were examined (see *Appendix 4*) by light microscopy under an oil immersion objective at x1000 magnification. Parasitaemia in thick blood film was estimated by counting parasite against leukocytes, 500 asexual forms or the number of parasites corresponding to 1000 leukocytes were counted whichever occurred first (Appendix 5).

Definition: The **parasite clearance time** was defined as the time from drug adminisration until there was no patent peripheral parasitaemia. The **fever clearance time** was defined as time from drug administration until the axillary temperature was 37.2°C or below and remains so far at least 72 hours. This definition was necessary because of the routine use of paracetamol during the first 36 h of treatment. The symptom clearance time was defined as the time between drug administration and the disappearance of all presenting symptoms. Classification of response to drug treatment was according to Sowunmi *et al*[81]. Treatment was considered a **failure** if parasitaemia on day 3 was greater than 25% of the day 0 value, if parasitaemia did not clear by Day 7, or if parasitaemia cleared before day 7 but re-appeared before day 14. The **cure rate** was defined as the proportion of children who remained free of parasitaemia on day 14 of follow-up[80]

All treatment failures were treated with the initial drug regimen on day 14 provided they were not symptomatic before this time. If they became symptomatic between day 7 and day 14, they were similarly treated. Patient with profound clinical symptoms (oral fluid intolerance, clouding of consciousness) during follow-up were started on intramuscular injection of artemether (3.2 mg/kg body weight) and referred to children emergency ward for further care.

Adverse drug reaction Monitoring

A specimen of adverse drug reaction form used during the study is shown in *Appendix 6* .Each patient, where possible, and/or parents were questioned in respect of the presenting symptoms and other symptoms that were noticed following institution of therapy. Appearance of new symptoms after commencement of drug administration was regarded as side effects of the drugs.

Statistical analysis

Data were analysed using *Epi-Info* version 6[82]. Proportions were compared by calculating chi square(x^2) with Yate's correction. Normally distributed data, for example, weight and temperature were compared by Student's t test. Data not conforming to normal distribution, for example, parasite density were compared by the Mann-Whitney's U test or the Kruskal-Walli's test. Values are given in the text (and tables) as mean $\pm$ standard deviation (sd). P values of less than 0.05 were taken as statistically significant.

Chart summary of activity

The chart summary of activity during the study is shown in Table 1.

Table 1: Chart summary of activity during the study

Activity	D0	D1	D2	D3	D4	D5	D6	D7	D14
Parasite identification & quantification.	x	x	x	x	x	x	x	x	x
History	x	x	x	x	x	x	x	x	x
Physical examination	x	x	x	x	x	x	x	x	x
Laboratory								x	
FBC	x							x	
Hb genotype	x							x	
G6PD	x							x	
Biochemistry	x							x	
Urine test									
Lignin	x								
Dill-Glazko	x								

Chapter 3

RESULTS

During the period of study (May - September 1998), a total of 132 patients aged 6 months - 14 years presented with symptoms suggestive of malaria. Of these, *P. falciparum* was demonstrated in blood smears of 113 (60 female and 53 males); a parasite rate of 85.6%.

Of the 113 children with *P.falciparum* parasitaemia; 105 of them were enrolled into the study having satisfied the enrolment criteria. Fifty-three of those enrolled were given chloroquine-chlorpheniramine while 52 children received halofantrine. The eighty-eight (47 females and 41 males) children that completed this study was evaluated. Forty-five of these children were in the chloroquine-chlorpheniramine group while 43 received halofantrine. Twenty-four and twenty-three females and, 21 and 20 males were given chloroquine-chlorpheniramine or halofantrine, respectively. Of those treated with chloroquine-chlorpheniramine one was discovered to have sickle cell anaemia and, even though successfully treated his data were excluded: the remaining 7 defaulted from the clinic mostly by days 3-5 of follow up, and all returned to the clinic after 3 weeks being symptomatic of malaria. Data of these children were also excluded in view of the violation of protocol. The 9 children in halofantrine group whose data were not included were as a result of ingestion of concomitant medication (cotrimoxazole) in 2 children, one child developed bronchopneumonia and was treated with amoxycillin-clavulanic acid while the remaining 6 defaulted on day two of follow up one of whom reported with symptomatic malaria on day 16 the others were not seen until 3 weeks later, also symptomatic of malaria.

Clinical features at presentation

The presenting symptoms of the children enrolled in (and completed) the study are shown in Table 2. The presenting symptoms were similar in the two groups. Fever was the commonest symptom at presentation, occurring in all the patients (100%). The other presenting symptoms were anorexia 10/88 (11.4%), abdominal pain14/88 (15.9%), headache 12/88 (13.6%), vomiting (21.2%), diarrhoea 6/88 (6.8%), cough 7/88 (8%) and lethargy 1/88(1.1%). The mean and median duration of illness was 3 days for the two treatment groups with range of 1-8 days for each group.

The clinical findings at presentation are shown in Table 3. These findings were similar in the two groups. The mean ages of chloroquine-chlorpheniramine group and halofantrine group were, respectively 6.5 ± 3.5 and 6.1 ± 3.8; P = 0.58. The mean weights of 18.3 ± 6.5 versus 16.9 ± 6.7 for the two treatment groups were also similar; P = 0.31. Also the mean temperature of $38.5^\circ C \pm 0.9$ in the chloroquine-chlorpheniramine group was similar to $37.9^\circ C \pm 3.2$; (P = 0.21) in the halofantrine group.

The mean heart rate in chloroquine-chlorpheniramine group was 117 ± 21 beats per minute and 119 ± 20 in the halofantrine group; the respiratory rate for the two groups were also similar, 33 cycles per minute and 34 cycles per minute for chloroquine-chlorpheniramine and halofantrine, respectively. Twenty-four and 23 children in the chloroquine - chlorpheniramine group and halofantrine group had hepatosplenomegaly: 11 and 9 respectively presented with enlarged liver only while 2 each were found to have splenic enlargement only.

Parasitological parameters of patients at enrolment

Table 4 shows anthropometric and parasitological findings at enrolment. The parasitological findings in the two groups were similar; the geometric mean parasite densities for chlorquine-chlorpheniramine and halofantrine were, respectively 34,536 vs 22,749 per microlitre of blood. Parasite density ranged between 1270 and 531,428/ul of blood for chloroquine-chlorpheniramine and 1149 and 1,842,000/ul of blood in the halofantrine group. There was no significant difference in the parasite densities in the two treatment groups.

Therapeutic Responses

Clearance of fever and other symptoms

Forty-one of of the children treated with chloroquine-chlorpheniramine were febrile at presentation (body temperature>37.2°C): 42 of those treated with halofantrine also had elevated temperature at presentation. In all these children temperature had become normalised by day 3 of follow up. The rate of clearance of fever in the two treatment groups was shown in Table 5. The rate of clearance of fever was similar in the two groups. The mean fever clearance times in chloroquine-chlorpheniramine group and halofantrine group were respectively 1.2$\pm$0.5 and 1.4$\pm$0.1 days. Figure 4 also shows that resolution of fever was similar in the two groups. Other presenting symptoms like anorexia, headache, and vomiting rapidly cleared in the patients such that by day 3, the symptoms had completely cleared in all the children.

Table 2: **Presenting symptoms of children with falciparum malaria treated with chloroquine- chlorpheniramine or halofantrine***

SYMPTOMS	Chloroquine-chlorpheniramine	Halofantrine	Total
Fever	45 (51.5)	43 (48.9)	88 (100)
Anorexia	6 (6.8)	4 (4.5)	10 (11.4)
Abdominal pain	8 (9.1)	6 (6.8)	14 (15.9)
Headache	10 (11.4)	2 (2.3)	12 (13.6)
Vomiting/Nausea	11 (12.5)	8 (9.1)	19 (21.6)
Diarrhoea	4 (4.5)	2 (2.3)	6 (6.8)
Cough	4 (4.5)	3 (3.4)	7 (8)
Lethargy/irritability	0 (0)	1 (1.1)	1 (1.1)

* Figures in the parenthesis are percentages

Table 3 Physical findings at enrolment of children with falciparum malaria treated with chloroquine-chlorpheniramine or halofantrine.

	Chloroquine-chlorpheniramine	Halofantrine
No of patients	45	43
Age(years)		
mean ± sd	6.5 ± 3.5	6.1 ± 3.8
range	0.8-13.7	0.8-13
Weight(kg)		
mean ± sd	18.3 ± 6.5	16.8 ± 6.7
range	9.0-34.0	6.5-32
Temperature(^{o}C)		
mean ± sd	38.5 ± 0.9	37.9 ± 3.2
range	36.6-40.4	36.5-40.4
Heart rate(beats/min)		
mean ± sd	117 ± 21	119 ± 20
range	76-168	80-160
Resp. rate(cycles/min)		
mean ± sd	33 ± 10	34 ± 11
range	18-64	14-60
Organ enlargement (no of patients)		
splenomegaly only	2	2
hepatomegaly only	11	9
hepatosplenomegaly	24	23

Table 4 Anthropometric and parasitological data of 88 children with falciparum malaria at enrolment

	Chloroquine-chlorpheniramine	Halofantrine
Number enrolled	n = 45	n = 43
Male:Female	21:24	20:23
Age (years)		
mean	6.5 ± 3.5	6.1 ± 3.8
range	0.8-13.7	0.8-13
Weight (kg)		
mean	18.3 ± 6.5	16.9 ± 6.7
range	9-34	6.5-32
Temperature oC		
mean	38.5 ± 0.9	37.9 ± 3.2
range	36.6-40.4	36.5-40.4
Parasite density (/ul)		
geometric mean	34,536	22,749
range	1270-531428	1149-1,842,000
no with >250,000/ul	3	2

Table 5 Rate of fever clearance in 83 children with documented elevated temperature at presentation a treated with chloroquine-chlorpheniramine and halofantrine

Day of follow up	Number of patients with temperature >37.2°C	
	Chloroquine-chlorpheramine	Halofantrine
0	41 (100%)	42 (100%)
1	9 (22%)	10 (23.8%)
2	2 (4.8%)	4 (9.5%)
3	0	0
4	0	0
5	0	0
6	0	0
7	0	0
Fever clearance time (days)		
mean ± sd	1.2 ± 0.5	1.4 ± 0.7 *
range	1-3	1-3

* $p = 0.23$

Clearance of parasitemia

Table 6 shows the rate of clearance of parasitaemia in the two treatment groups. The proportion of patients in whom parasitaemia cleared on days 2 and 3 of follow up were similar: 13/45 (28.95) and 14/43 (32.6%) in the chloroquine-chlorpheniramine and halofantrine groups, respectively on day 2, and 33/45 (73.3%) and 31/43 (72.1%) in the chloroquine -chlorpheniramine group and halofantrine group, respectively on day 3. However, on days 4, 5 and 6 parasitaemia was still present in 7, 1 and 1 patients, respectively in the chloroquine-chlorpheniramine. The mean parasite clearance time was significantly shorter in the halofantrine group than the chloroquine-chlorpheniramine (2.3 ± 0.5 and 2.8$\pm$0.7 days, p = 0.001). Figure 5 shows the rate of clearance of parasitaemia in the two groups. The recurrence of parasitaemia was similar in the two treatment groups (Table 7). R1 type responses were seen in 2 patients each in the chloroquine-chlorpheniramine group and halofantrine group. One R11 type response was seen in the chloroquine-chlorpheniramine group. No patient had R111 type responseto therapy in the two treatment groups. The clinical and parasitological features of the treatment failures from both groups are summarized in Table 8. These features were similar in the two groups.

Adverse effects of treatment

The adverse effeccts of treatment in the two treatment groups are shown on Table 9. Pruritus was the most commonly reported side effect in chloroquine-chlorpheniramine group, occuring in 9 (20%) of the children, while abdominal pain with diarrhoea was the most commonly reported adverse effect in the halofantrine group. Pruritus was mild in all cases, occurred between days 1 and 3 and lasted for less than 72 hours in all children reporting this adverse effect in the chloroquine-chlorpheniramine group. Pruritus also occurred in one patient treated with halofantrine on day 1 of follow up. It was mild and lasted for less than 48 hours. In the four children reporting abdominal pain with diarrhoea on day 1 of follow up in the halofantrine group this adverse effect was mild and lasted for less than 24 hours. Abdominal pain and or diarrhoea did not occur in any patient in the choroquine-chlorpheniramine group.

41

Table 6 Rate of clearance of peripheral parasitaemie in 88 children treated with chloroquine-chlorpheniramine or halofantrine

	Number of patients with peripheral parasitaemia	
Day	Chloroquine-chlorpheniramine	Halofantrine
0	45 (100%)	43 (100%)
1	45 (100%)	43 (100%)
2	32 (71.1)	29 (67.4)
3	12 (26.7%)	12 (27.9%)
4	7 (15.6%)	0
5	1 (2.2%)	0
6	1 (2.2%)	0
7	3 (6.7%)	2 (4.7%)
14	3 (6.7%)	2 (4.7%)
Parasite clearance time(days)	2.8 ± 0.7	2.3 ± 0.5 *
Mean	2-5	2-4
Range	93.3	95.3**
Parasitological cure rate(%)		

* $p = 0.001$
** $p = 0.9$

Table 7: Response to chloroquine-chlorpheniramine and halofantrine in 88 children treated for falciparum malaria

	Chloroquine-chlorpheniramine	Halofantrine
No of patients	45	43
M:F	21:24	20:23
Age(years)		
mean	6.5±3.5	6.1± 3.8
range	0.8-13.7	0.8-13
FCT (days)		
mean	1.2 ± 0.5	1.4± 0.7 *
range	1-3	1-3
PCT (days)		
mean	2.8 ± 0.7	2.3± 0.5 **
range	2-5	2-4
Response		
cure rate day 14 (%)	93.3	95.3***
Treatment failure (no of patiens)		
R1	2	2
R11	1	0
R111	0	0

FCT   Fever clearance time

PCT   parasite clearance time

*   p=0.23

**   P=0.001

***   p=0.9

Table 8 Pre-treatment anthropometric and parasitological features of chloroquine-chlorpheniramine or halofantrine treatment failures

	Chloroquine-chlorpheniramine	Halofantrine
No of patients	3	2
sex: F:M	2:1	1:1
Age (years)		
mean $\pm$ sd	2.2 $\pm$ 0.6	2.0 $\pm$ 1.0
range	1.67-3	1.1-3
Duration of illness (days)		
mean $\pm$ sd	3 $\pm$ 0.8	2.5 $\pm$ 0.5
range	2-4	2-3
weight (kg)		
mean $\pm$ sd	10.6 $\pm$ 2.1	11.6 $\pm$ 3.0
range	9-13.5	8.6-14.5
Temperature (^{O}C)		
mean $\pm$ sd	38.8 $\pm$ 0.8	39 $\pm$ 0.6
range	38.2-39.9	38.4-39.6
Parasite density (/ul)		
geometric mean	36890	101826
range	2880-391200	5629-1842000

44

Table 9: Adverse effects of Chloroquine-chlorpheniramine and halofantrine in children with acute falciparum malaria*

	Chloroquine-chlorpheniramine	Halofantrine
No of Patients	45	43
Pruritus	9 (20)	1 (2.3)
Abdominal pain	0-	4 (9.3)
Drowsiness	1 (2.2)	0
Diarrhoea	0	2 (4.7)
Haemogblobinuria	0	1 (2.3)

*Figures in the parenthesis are percentages

One 12 year old boy in the halofantrine group had intravascular haemolysis characterised by dark coloured urine (haemoglobinuria) and marked drop in haematocrit on day 2 of treatment. (haematocrit at enrolment was 34% and 24% on day 2). This child appeared very ill on day 2 with body temperature of 37.8°C,a packed cell volume of 24% and normal Glucose 6 phosphate dehydrogenase enzyme activiy (sample collected at enrolment). There was a mild increase in plasma creatinine from 0.9 mg on day 0 but 1.1 mg per decilitre on day 2. He was kept in the clinic for 6 hours during which he was rehydrated by oral route and was only allowed home after improvement was noticed. He remained well throughout the period of follow-up.

Tolerance (and safety)

Pulse

At enrolment, the pulse rate of the children was above normal (Table 3). By day 3 the pulse rate had returned to normal and remained within normal range throughout the period of follow up (Table 10). The rates were regular and similar in the two treatment groups during the entire period of the study (Table 10 & Figure 6). No child developed bradycardia (heart rate <60/min) during the entire period of the study.

Blood pressure

The systolic and diastolic blood pressure recordings at enrolment and at follow up in the two groups are shown in Table 11 and Figures 7a & b. The values at enrolment and during follow up were similar in the two groups. In addition, the values during follow up were not significantly different from those at enrolment (ANOVA: $F = 012$, $p = 0.99$, systolic); ($F = 0.75$, $p = 0.65$, diastolic) for chloroquine-chlorpheniramine, and ANOVA for halofantrine group systolic and diastolic blood pressure were, respectively $F = 0.37$, $p = 0.94$ and $F = 0.12$, $p = 0.99$ (Table 11).

46

Respiratory rate

The respiratory rates at enrolment and during follow up in the two groups are shown in Table 12 and Figure 8. In general, the rates at enrolment and during the first two days after enrolment were higher than on subsequent days. However, the rates at all times were similar in the two treatment groups. No abnormal pattern of respiration was encountered at enrolment and during follow up.

Body temperature

Group mean body temperature at enrolment and during follow-up was similar in the two groups (Table 13). Group mean body temperature which was raised in both groups at enrolment normalised by day 1 and remained within normal limits throughout the study. Hypothermia was not encountered in any child during follow up period.

Table 10 Group mean pulse rate (beats/min) at enrolment and during follow up in the children with falciparum malaria treated with chloroquine-chlorpheniramine or halofantrine

	Chloroquine-chlorpheniramine (n=45)	Halofantrine (n=43)	p values
Day 0			
mean$\pm$ sd	117$\pm$ 21	119 $\pm$20	p=0.6
range	76-168	80-160	
Day 1			
mean$\pm$ sd	103$\pm$ 21	105$\pm$20	p=0.68
range	72-156	76-156	
Day 2			
mean +/-sd	109$\pm$ 21	108+/- 21	p=0.82
range	70-140	76-140	
Day 3			
mean $\pm$sd	90 $\pm$15	90 $\pm$ 14	p=0.95
range	72-132	72-116	
Day 4			F=0.27, p=0.60
mean$\pm$ sd	86$\pm$ 11	87 $\pm$ 11	
rRange	70-104	72-124	
Day 5			
mean$\pm$sd	86$\pm$ 10	89$\pm$ 12	p=0.15
range	72-102	72-120	
Day 6			
mean $\pm$sd	88$\pm$ 10	88$\pm$10	p=0.92
range	80-120	76-104	
Day 7			
mean$\pm$ sd	93$\pm$10	91$\pm$ 10	0.21
range	68-112	72-104	
Day 14			
mean $\pm$sd	93$\pm$9	90$\pm$10	p=0.22
range	72-104	72-100	

Figure 6

Table 11 Systolic and diastolic blood pressure in children with falciparum malaria treated
with chloroquine-chlorpheniramine or halofantrine*

	Chloroquine-chlorpheniramine n = 45	Halofantrine n = 43	p values
D0			
mean ±sd	SBP 87.3 ±15.6	SBP 86 ±10.7	p=0.65
range	80-110	80-110	
mean ±	DBP 50.4 ±11.4	DBP 49.3±10.3	p=0.63
range	40-70	40-70	
D1			
mean ±sd	SBP 88.5 ± 15.1	SBP 88.9±10.9	p=0.89
range	70-120	70-110	
mean ±sd	DBP 50.3±11.3	DBP 49.7± 10.7	p=0.80
range	40-70	40-70	
D2			
mean ± sd	SBP 87.9±15.3	SBP 86.1±10.9	p=0.53
range	70-120	70-118	
mean ± sd	DBP 52.1±14.7	DBP 50 ± 11.3	p=0.46
range	48-80	44-76	
D3			
mean ± sd	SBP 87.1±15.1	SBP 85.9±11.5	p=0.68
range	70-110	70-110	
mean± sd	DBP 51.9±11.9	DBP 50.1±11.1	p=0.47
range	40-70	46-76	
D7			
mean ± sd	SBP 88.2± 8.1	SBP 87.2±9.6	p=0.6
range	80-110	80-120	
mean ± sd	DBP 52± 7.2	DBP 50.9 ± 10	p=0.55
range	40-70	40-70	
D14			
mean ± sd	SBP 89.1± 7.0	SBP 87.7± 9.8	p=0.44
range	80-110	80-110	
mean ± sd	DBP 50.7±7.1	DBP 49.1 ± 9.7	p=0.38
range	50-76	50-80	

** SBP-systolic blood pressure (mmHg)
  DBP-diastolic blood pressure (mmHg)
*All measurements were taken in supine position

Table 12 Respiratory rate (cycles/minute) before and after treatment treated with chloroquine-chlorpheniramine or halofantrine in children with acute falciparum malaria

	Chloroquine-chlorpheniramine (n=45)	Halofantrine (n=43)	p values
D0			
mean ±sd	32.6 ± 10.3	34.4± 11.4	p=0.44
range	18-64	14-60	
D1			
mean ± sd	30.8 ± 9.5	31.1 ± 10.2	p=0.89
range	18-56	14-56	
D2			
mean ±sd	31.6 ± 9.7	29.6 ± 10.1	p=0.35
range	18-56	14-48	
D3			
mean ± sd	20.9 ± 5.7	19.1 ±5.3	p=0.13
range	18-36	16-32	
D4			
mean ±sd	21.5± 4.9	20.3±4.3	p=0.23
range	16-40	14-34	
D5			
mean ±sd	19.4 ± 4.7	18.7 ± 4.2	p=0.46
range	16-40	14-36	
D6			
mean ±sd	20.1 ± 4.5	19.4 ± 4.1	p=0.49
range	16-36	14-28	
D7			
mean ±sd	21.9 ± 4.3	20.7 ± 3.7	p=0.16
range	16-32	14-28	
D14			
mean ±sd	21.5 ±4.0	21.1 ±3.9	p=0.64
range	16-32	14-30	

Table 13 Group mean temperature ($^{\circ}$C) in children with falciparum malaria treated with chlorquine-chlorpheniramine or halofantrine

	Chloroquine-chlorpheniramine (n=45)	Halofantrine (n=43)	p values
D0			
mean ± sd	38.5 ± 1.0	38.4 ± 0.8	p=0.60
range	36.5-40.4	36.-40.4	
D1			*
mean ±sd	36.9 ± 0.9	36.9±0.7	
range	36-39.1	36.2-39.1	
D2			
mean ±sd	36.5 ±0.5	36.7 ± 0.5	p=0.10
range	35.9-37.5	35.9-39.9	
D3			
mean ±sd	36.4± 0.4)	36.3± 0.4	p=0.27
range	35.9-37.2	36.0-37.1	
D4			
mean ±sd	36.5± 0.4	36.4±0.4	p=0.23
range	35.9-37.1	36-37	
D5			
mean ±sd	36.3±0.4	36.4±0.4	p=0.21
range	35.9-37	36.0-37.0	
D6			
mean ±sd	36.4±0.4	36.3±0.4	p=0.24
range	36-37	36.0-37.0	
D7			
mean ±sd	36.3±0.4	36.5±0.3	p=0.18
range	35.9-37	35.9-37.1	
D14			
mean ±sd	36.5±0.4	36.4±0.4	p=0.20
range	35.9-37.0	36.0-37.0	

*   Equal means

Laboratory parameters

Haematology

Anaemia was the commonest haematological disorder found. The haematocrit at presentation was less than 30% in 38 (48%) patients (Table 14). When compared, haematocrit at enrolment was not statistically different in both (treatment) groups, thus haematocrit in the chloroquine-chlorpheniramine group and halofantrine pre-treatment were 30±4.8% and 28.1±5.3%, p>0.05. Also no significant difference was found when proportion of patients aged 5 years and below with haematocrit < 30% was compared with the others 53.8% and 38.2%, P=0.23.

The total white cell count was similar pre-treatment in the two groups 6073 ± 1715 and 5740 ±1415 per cubic mm in the chloroquine-chlorpheniramine group and halofantrine groups, respectively. Comparison of the total white cell count pre- and post-treatment did not reveal any significant difference 5851±1615 and 5925 ± 1472; p=0.41). The mean neutrophil count was wthin normal limits pre treatment in the two groups. At presentation, mean monocyte count of the children treated with chloroquine chlopheniramine and halofantrine were 216 ± 120 and 133 ± 58, respectively. The monocyte count on day 7 for both treatment groups were 73 ± 33 and 103 ±67 monocytes per cubic millimeter.

Blood Biochemistry:

The tables 15 & 16 show the results of the biochemical parameters of the children before and after treatment in the two groups. The values were within normal limits and similar in the two treatment groups. These values were similar before and after treatment in the two groups. In addition, the values were not significantly different in the two groups.

Table 14: Haematological parameters of children with acute falciparum malaria pre- and post-treatment with chloroquine-chlorpheniramine or halofantrine

	Chloroquine-chlorpheniramine		Halofantrine	
PCV (%)	day 0 (n=40)	day 7 (n=33)	day 0 (n=39)	day 7 (n=28)
mean ± sd	30±4.8	29.2 ± 4	28.1 +/- 5.3	27.9 ± 5.2
range	18-40	20-34	17-36	17-34
No with PCV				
<30%	18	17	22	19
WBC (/mm³)				
mean±sd	6073±1715	5816±1615	5740±1415	5630±1458
range	3500-11200	3500-8100	2200-13000	3200-9300
Neutrophil (/mm³)				
mean ±sd	4097±1643	3511±1827	3369±1345	3616±1009
Range	1386-4221	1952-5184	1144-4952	1180-5544
Monocyte (/mm³)				
mean ±sd	216±120	73±33	133±58	103±67
range	0-475	0-189	0-236	0-215
Lymphocyte. (/mm³)				
mean ±sd	1806±1710	2014±1542	2287±1847	2315±1799
range	1190-3920	1247-3205	1220-4025	1219-3618

54

Table 15 Blood electrolytes and creatinine of children with falciparum malaria pre- and post-treatment with chloroquine-chlorpheniramine or halofantrine

	Chloroquine-chlorpheniramine		Halofantrine	
Sodium	day 0 n=33	day 7 n=32	day 0 n=34	day 7 n=33
(mmol/L)				
mean±sd	139.9±4.5	140±6.3	140±4.6	140±6.2
range	130-152	121-152	130-154	124-150
Potassium				
(mmol/L)				
mean±sd	3.4±0.3	4.0±0.5	3.6±0.4	3.9±0.4
range	2.9-4.5	3.2-5.4	3.1-4.8	3.2-4.6
Chloride				
(mmol/L)				
mean±sd	98.3 ± 7.3	101.4 ± 7.2	98.4 ± 7.7	101.3±7
range	85-115	85-116	85-112	86-115
Bicarbonate				
(mmol/L)				
mean ± sd	22.3 ±3.6	22.7 ± 3.0	22.4± 3.7	22.6 ± 2.9
range	15-29	18-28	15-29	19-28
Creatinine				
(mg/dL)				
mean ±sd	0.9 ±0.2	1.0 ± 0.2	1.0 ± 0.2	1.0 ±0.2
range	0.9-1.4	0.7-1.4	0.9-1.3	0.7-1.3

16 Liver function tests in children with acute malaria before and after treatment with chloroquine-chlorpheniramine or halofantrine

	Chloroquine-chlorpheniramine		Halofantrine	
	day 0 n=33	day 7 n=32	day 0 n=34	day 7 n=33
Bilirubin (mg/dL)				
mean±sd	0.4 ± 0.1	0.4 ± 0.1	0.4 ± 0.1	0.4+0.1
range	0.3-0.5	0.3-0.5	0.3-0.5	0.3-0.5
AST (i.u/L)				
mean±sd	27 ± 15.2	30.3 ± 14.1	28.9 ± 15.8	30.4 ± 14.0
range	10-83	12-58	12-93	13-54
ALT(i.u/l/L)				
mean±sd	24.7± 14.4	25.3 ± 10.7	25.1 ± 15.1	24.9±10.1
range	8-73	10-48	10-69	10-47
ALP (i.u/L)				
mean±sd	209 ± 122	205± 78	207 ± 123	205 ± 77
range	85-594	80-370	86-585	89-330
Total protein(g/L)				
mean±sd	6.1 ± 1.4	6.7 ± 1.0	6.0 ± 1.3	6.8 ± 1.1
range	3.4-9	4.6-8.4	3.5-8.5	4.2-8.1
Albumin (g/L)				
mean±sd	3.2± 0.8	3.6± 0.8	3.3 ± 0.7	3.6 ± 0.7
range	1.3-4.9	2.3-5.2	2.1-4.7	2.4-5.1

Chapter 4

DISCUSSION

In this study, all the children presented with symptoms compatible with acute uncomplicated falciparum malaria. All had fever but only about 20% presented with vomiting. None vomited the treatment drugs. None of the patients presented with unusual symptoms of malaria such as urinary frequency, psychosis or mononeuritis multiplex[10]. Abdominal organ enlargement was commonly found at examination; 58% and 73% of the children had splenomegaly and hepatomegaly respectively at presentation. The spleen rate of 58% suggests that the area is hyperendemic for malaria[83], although this figure was derived from symptomatic cases. The fact that hepatomegaly was more commonly found than splenomegaly in this endemic area suggests that the enlargement of the former may serve as a malariometric index[84], but this suggestion would need confirmation in carefully designed epidemiological studies. The liver rate of 73% is in agreement with that of similar study from the same area[84].

The response to treatment in the two groups was comparable. The fever clearance times in the chloroquine- chlorpheniramine and halofantrine groups were 1.2 and 1.4 days, respectively. The similar fever clearance times are comparable to those obtained from previous studies of chloroquine -chlorpheniramine and halofantrine from the same area of Nigeria[35 80]. The values are also similar to those for other drugs such as mefloquine, mefloquine-sulphadoxine-pyrimethamine, and chloroquine (in sensitive strains) from the same area of Nigeria[22 28].

Despite similar parasite densities at enrolment, parasite clearance time was significantly shorter in the halofantrine group than in the chloroquine-chlorpheniramine group. However, the cure rates on day 14 were similar. The reason(s) for the slower parasite clearance in the chloroquine chlorpeniramine group is (are) not readily apparent from the results of the present study. It is, however, possible that the slower parasite clearance may, perhaps be a

57

result of the relatively reduced sensitvity to chloroquine in the area[63]. In this regard, the enhancement of the antimalaria effect of chloroquine by chlorpheniramine may have led to eventual (but slow) clearance of those chloroquine resistant stains[63]. An *in vitro* sensitivity study, and its correlation with *in vivo* response in the same patients would have shed more light on this aspect of the enhancement of the efficacy of chloroquine by chlorpheniramine as was previously done in the same area of study[63].

When compared with a similar study from the same area[63] the cure rate for chloroquine-chlorpheniramine on day 14 in the present study was relatively higher (85% vs 93.3%) The reasons for this apparently higher cure rate may be due to (1) the fact that a higher dose of chlorpheniramine was used in the present study. Thus it is possible that chlorpheniramine induced reversal of chloroquine resistance in falciparum malaria infections may be chlorpheniramine dose-related, and (2) a higher dose of chloroquine was used in the present study (30 mg/kg compared to 25 mg/kg body weight). The cure rate, however, is similar to that from a recent study in which the same doses of chloroquine plus chlorpheniramine were used[80]. The higher dose of chloroquine used has been recomended for treatment of malaria in some other parts of the West-Africa sub-region, for example, The Gambia[85].

There has been a progressive decline in the sensitivity of *P. falciparum* to chloroquine in Southwest Nigeria; the cure rate was 75-80% in 1990, 85% in 1992 and 45-55% in 1997[22, 24, 27]. The cure rate of 93% in the children treated with chloroquine plus chlorpheniramine in the present study would suggest some efficacy of the combination in chloroquine resistant malaria.

Adverse reactions encountered in the study were, in general, mild and did not necessitate discontinuation of drug treatment in either treatment group. Pruritus was the most commonly reported adverse effect in children treated with chloroquine plus chlorpheniramine. This adverse effect occurred in 20% of the children. This high rate of pruritus despite addition of chlorpheniramine, would suggest the lack of effect of chlorpheniramine in reducing

58

chloroquine-induced pruritus in children. Pruritus was relatively uncommon in children treated with halofantrine. The low rate (2%) in this study is considerably lower than 13% previously reported for halofantrine in the same area[26][35]. The reason(s) for the low rate of pruritus is (are) unclear, but it is possible that under-reporting or documentation may occur in children. A potentially serious adverse effect seen with halofatrine but not with the combination was intravascular haemolysis which occurred in a 12 year old boy who had normal G-6-PD enzyme activity. This relatively serious adverse effect of halofantrine should be carefully watched for in patients treated with this drug. The absence of intravascular haemolysis in those treated with chloroquine plus chlorpheniramine may be an advantage over halofantrine. Both halofantrine and chloroquine may have deleterious cardiac effects[76][77]. The most common cardiac effects of both drugs is the prolonged rate corrected (QTc) interval on the electrocardiogram. Sudden death may occur after halofantrine therapy and is attributable to the development of cardiac arrhythmias[76, 77] following prolonged QTc interval. Chloroquine may also cause sudden death particularly after parenteral injections[68, 69]. Although, electrocardiographic monitoring was not done in any of children studied, none of the children presented with symptoms or signs suggestive of undue deleterious cardiac effects of both drugs. Recent studies (Sowunmi, unpublished data) have shown that both halofatrine and chloroquine equally prolong the QTc intervals in children suffering from acute uncomplicated falciparum malaria. However, P-R interval while being greatly prolonged by halofantrine, is relatively unaffected by chloroquine. The addition of chlorpheniramine to chloroquine also insignificantly amplified the QTc prolongation by chloroquine, but has no effect on P-R interval (Sowunmi, unpublished). It is, however, important to monitor carefully the cardiovascular system in patients treated with both drugs.

Anaemia (haematocrit<30%) was present in 50% of the children at enrolment. The anaemia of malaria is multifactorial; haemolytic destruction of parasitised red blood cells and dyserythropoiesis are contributory[26, 86, 87]. In addition, children in poor endemic countries may have poor nutritional status and may harbour helminthic infections which may cause anaemia. After treatment anaemia was still present in almost the same proportion of children as at presentation. The slow recovery from anaemia is not unusual at 1 or 2 weeks after treatment, but rapid increase in packed cell volume is seen by the end of the third week.

Other haematological parameters were not adversely affected by the two drugs (Table 14). It is particularly noteworthy that neutropenia/leukopenia was not seen in any of the children treated with chloroquine plus chlorpheniramine; chlorpheniramine may occasionally cause neutropenia. In addition, none of the children presented with symptoms suggestive of infections which may be attributable to neutropenia.

Biochemical parameters monitored during the studies were not adversely affected by both treatment regimens. In addition, the parameters were similar in both treatment groups. Both drugs may cause mild increase in liver enzymes, but this is commoner with halofantrine[27]. Although serum creatinine concentrations were wthin normal limits in all the children, recent studies indicate that biochemical evidence of renal function impairment are not uncommon in children with acute uncomplicated falciparum malaria. The impaired renal function may persist for a variable period of time after complete clearance of peripheral parasitaemia and full clinical recovery. In addition symptoms suggestive of renal function impairment are not usually seen in this group of children[88].

Although the combination of chloroquine plus chlorpheniramine is effective in this area with moderate chloroquine resistance, the exact mechanism(s) for the reversal of chloroquine resistance in *P. falciparum* by chlorpeniramine is (are) unknown[63]. Reversal is only seen in resistant but not sensitive strains[59, 63], and is related to the reduced efflux of chloroquine by the resistant strains[55]. However, chlorpheniramine may increase the peak plasma chloroquine concentrations and area under the plasma concentration time curve (AUC) after co-administration (with chloroquine) to healthy individuals[89]. This phenomenon, if it occurs in acute malaria may possibly contribute to the enhancement of the efficacy of chloroquine by chlorpheniramine. Certainly, detailed pharmacokinetic and pharmacodynamics studies are needed to determine the mechanism(s) of the enhanced efficacy of chlorpheniramine-chloroquine combination in falciparum malaria.

CONCLUSION

The present study has shown that

1. The combination of chloroquine and chlorpheniramine is effective in falciparum malaria in children in an area where the reported rate of chloroquine resistance is 35-45%.

2. The combination of chloroquine plus chlorpheniramine is as effective as halofantrine, a drug used in the treatment of chloroquine resistant falciparum malaria, in the treatment of falciparum malaria in children from an endemic area.

3. Chloroquine plus chlorpheniramine and halofantrine are safe and well tolerated by a group of children with falciparum malaria resident in an endemic area.

RECOMMENDATIONS

It is recommended that

1. More studies should be carried out in many endemic areas to confirm the effectiveness of chloroquine-chlorpheniramine in chloroquine resistant malaria.

2. Studies to correlate *in vitro* with *in vivo* sensitivity of *P. falciparum* to the combination of chloroquine plus chlorpheniramine be done in the same patients.

3. Detailed pharmacokinetic studies be done to elucidate the interactions of chloroquine with chlorpheniramine in healthy subjects and in patients with malaria.

4. More studies on the pharmacokinetic, pharmacodynamic and molecular basis of reversal be undertaken in order to elucidate the mechanism(s) of reversal of chloroquine resistance in *P. falciparum* by chlorpheniramine.

LIMITATION OF THE STUDY

1.   The treatment failures estimation of drug concentrations in biological fluids should have been done in order to confirm absorption or otherwise of the drugs.

2.   An *in vitro/ in vivo* correlation study should have been done in the same set of treatment failures, and in randomly selected patients in the chloroquine-chlorpheniramine group.

References

1. WHO. World Malaria situation in 1989 Part I. Weekly Epidimiological Record. 1991; 66: 157-163.

2. Lepes T. Present status of the global malaria eradication programme and prospects for the future. J Trop Med Hyg. 1974; 77: 47-53.

3. Nigeria Federal Ministry of Health. Guidelines for malaria control in Nigeria. July 1989.

4. Gilles HM, Warrell DA. Pathology and pathophysiology of human malaria, In: Bruce-Chwatt's Essential Malariology 3rd Edition, Great Britain: Edward Arnold. 1993: pp.50-56.

5. Salako LA, Ajayi FO, Sowunmi A, Walker O. Malaria in Nigeria: a revisit. Ann Trop Med Parasitol.1990; 84: 435-445.

6. WhiteNJ, Plorde J. In: Harrison's Principles of Internal Medicine McGraw-Hill Inc. New York. 12th edition 1991: Pp 782-788.

7. Krotoski WA. Discovery of the hypnozoite and a new theory of malarial relapse. Trans R Soc Trop Med Hyg. 1985; 79:1-11.

8. Rajan TV. Why does Plasmodium have a pre-erythrocytic cycle? Parasitol Today 1997; 13: 284-287.

9. Godfrey-Faussett P, Behrens RH, Kapoor R. Mononeuritis multiplex in *Plasmodium falciparum* malaria. Trans R Soc Trop Med Hyg 1990; 84: 351-352.

10. Sowunmi A, Ohaeri JU, Falade CO. Falciparum malaria presenting as psychosis. Trop Geog Med 1995; 47: 218-219.

11. Petersen E, Marbiah NT. QBC(R) and thick blood films for malaria diagnosis under field conditions. Trans R Soc Trop Med Hyg 1994; 88: 416-417.

12. Oduola AMJ, Omitowoju GO, SowunmiA, Makler MT, Falade CO Kyle DE, Fehintola FA, Ogundahunsi OAT, Piper RC, Schuster BG, Milhous WK. *Plasmodium falciparum*: Evaluation of lactate dehydrogenase in monitoring therapeutic responses to standard Antimalarial Drugs in Nigeria. Expt Parasitol 1997; 87: 283-289.

13. Knobloch J, Henk M. Screening for malaria by determination of parasite specific lactate dehydrogenase. Trans R Soc Trop Med Hyg 1995; 89: 269-270.

14. Premji Z, Minjas JN, Shiff CJ. Laboratory diagnosis of malaria by village health workers using the rapid manual parasight TM-F test.Trans R Soc Trop Med Hyg 1994; 88: 418.

15. Ezedinachi E. In vivo efficacy of chloroquine, halofantrine, pyrimethamine-sulphadoxine and qinghaosu in the treatment of malaria in Calabar, Nigeria. Cent Afr J Med 1996; 42: 109-111.

16. Wernsdorfer WH. The development and spread of drug-resistant malaria. Parasitology Today 1991; 7: 297-303.

17. Fogh S, Jepsen S, Effersoe P. Chloroquine resistant *Plasmodium falciparum* malaria in Kenya. Trans R Soc Trop Med Hyg 1979; 73: 228-229.

18. Weniger BG, Blumberg RS, Campbell CC, Jones TC, Mount DL, Friedman SM. High-lvevel chloroquine resistance of *Plasmodium falciparum* malaria acquired in Kenya. New Engl J Med. 1982; 307: 1560-1562.

19. Ekanem OJ, Weisfeld JS, Salako LA, Nahlen BL, Ezedinachi ENU, Walker O, Breman JG, Laoye OJ, Hedberg K. Sensitivity of *Plasmodium falciparum* to chloroquine and sulphadoxine-pyrimethamine in Nigerian children. Bull Wld Hlth Org. 1990; 68: 45-52.

20. WHO. Advances in Malaria Chemotherapy. Geneva: World Health Organization, Technical Report Series. 1984; No. 711 Pp 1-101.

21. Hatton C, PetoT, Bunch C, Pasvol G, Russell S, Singer C, Edwards G, Winstanley P. Frequency of severe neutropenia associated with amodiaquine prophylaxis against malaria. Lancet. 1986; 1: 411-413.

22. Sowunmi A, Salako LA. Evaluation of the relative efficacy of various antimalarial drugs in Nigerian children under five years of age suffering from acute uncomplicated falciparum malaria. Ann Trop Med Parasitol 1992; 86: 1-8.

23. Sowunmi A, Akindele JA, Omitowoju GO, Omigbodun AO, Oduola AMJ, Salako LA. Intramuscular sulphadomine-pyrimathemine in uncomplicated chloroquine-resistant falciparum malaria during pregnancy. Trans R Soc Trop Med Hyg 1993; 87: 472-473.

24. Adagu IS, Warhurst DC, Ogala WN, Abdu-Aguye I, Audu LI, Bamgbola FO, Ovwigho UB. Antimalarial drug response of *Plasmodium falciparum* from Zaria, Nigeria. Trans R Soc Med Hyg 1995; 89: 422-425.

25. OlatundeA SalakoLA WalkerO. The *in vivo* sensitivity of *Plasmodium falciparum* to chloroquine and sulphadoxine pyrimethamine combination in Ibadan. Nigeria. Trans R Soc Trop Med Hyg. 1981; 75: 848-850.

26. WHO. Severe and Complicated malaria. Trans R Soc Trop Med Hyg 1990; 84: Supplement 2, 1-65.

27. Falade CO, Salako LA, Sowunmi A, Oduola AMJ, Lacier P. Comparative efficacy of halofantrine, chloroquine and sulphadoxine-pyrimethamine in treatment of acute uncomplicated falciparum malaria in Nigerian children. Trans R Soc Trop Med Hyg 1997; 91: 58-62.

28. Sowunmi A, Oduola AMJ. Open comparison of chloroquine, mefloquine, mefloquine/sulfadoxine/pyrimethamine in acute uncomplicated falciparum malaria in children. Trans R Soc Trop Med Hyg 1995; 89: 303-305.

29. Karbwang T, Bangchang K, Thanavibul A, Bunnag D, Chongsulphajaisiddhi T, Harrinasuta T. Comparison of oral artemether and mefloquine in acute uncomplicated falciparum malaria. Lancet. 1992; 86: 123-126.

30. Sowunmi A, Salako LA, Oduola AMJ, Walker O, Akindele JA, Ogundahunsi OAT. Neuropsychiatric side effects of mefloquine in Africans. Trans R Soc Trop Med Hyg. 1993; 87: 462-463.

31. Oduola AMJ, Sowunmi A, Milhous WK, Kyle DE, Martin RK, Walker O, Salako LA. Innate resistance to new antimalarial drugs in *Plasmodium falciparum* from Nigeria. Trans R Soc Trop Med Hyg 1992; 86: 123-126.

32. Desjardins RE, Canfield CJ, Haynes JD, Chulay JD. Quantitative assessment of antimalaria activity in vitro by a semiautomated microdilution technique. Antimicrobial Agents and Chemotherapy. 1979; 16: 710-718.

33. Karbwang J, Milton KA, Na Bangchang K, Ward SA, Edwards G, Bunnag D. Pharmacokinetics of halofantrine in Thai patients with acute uncomplicated falciparum malaria. Br J Clin Pharmac.1991; 31, 484-487.

34. Milton KA EdwardsG WardSA Orme ME Breckenridge AM. Pharmacokinetics of halofantrine in man: Effects of food and dose size. Br J Clin Pharmac. 1989; 28: 71-77.

35. Salako LA, Sowunmi A, Walker O. Evaluation of the clinical efficacy and safety of halofantrine in falciparum malaria in Ibadan, Nigeria. Trans R Soc Trop Med Hyg 1990; 84: 644-647.

36. Hall AP. The treatment of malaria. Br Med J. 1976; 1:323-328.

37. WHO. Chemotherapy of Malaria and Resistance to antimalarials. Report of a WHO Scientific Group. Technical Report Series 1973; no 529 Pp 1-78.

38. Spencer HC. Drug-resistant malaria: Changing patterns mean difficult decisions. Trans R Soc Trop Med Hyg 1985; 79: 748-758.

39. Wernsdorfer WH. Drug resistant malaria. Endeavour New Series 1984; 8(4): 166-171.

40. Peters W. The problem of drug resistance in malaria. Parasitology 1985; 90: 705-715.

41. Hien TT, White NJ. Qinghaosu. Lancet 1993; 341: 603-8.

42. Myint PT, Shwe T. A controlled clinical trial of artemether (quinghaosu derivative) versus quinine in complicated and severe falciparum malaria. Trans R Soc Trop Med Hyg.1987; 81: 559-561.

43. Tongyin W, Ruchang X. Clinical studies of treatment of falciparum malaria with artemether, a derivative of qinghaosu. J Trad Chinese Med 1985; 5: 240-242.

44. Sowunmi A, Oduola AMJ. Artemether treatment of recrudescent *Plasmodium falciparum* malaria in children. Trop Med Int Health 1997; 2: 631-634.

45. Sowunmi A, Oduola AMJ, Salako LA. Artemether treatment of sulfadoxine-pyrimethamine-resistant *Plasmodium falciparum* malaria in children. Trans R Soc Trop Med Hyg 1995; 89: 435-436.

46. Sowunmi A, Oduola AMJ, Ogundahunsi OAT, Fehintola FA, Ilesanmi OA, Akinyinka OO, ArowojoluAO. Randomised trial of artemether vs artemether and mefloquine for treatment of chloroquine,sulphadoxine-pyrimethamine resistant falciparum malaria during pregnancy. J Obst Gynaecol. 1998;18:322-327

47. Price RN, Nosten F, Luxemburger C, et al. Artesunate versus artemether in combination with mefloquine for the treatment of multidrug resistant falciparum malaria. Trans R Soc Trop Med Hyg. 1995; 89: 523-527.

48. WhiteNJ. Artemisinin: current status. Trans R Soc Trop Med Hyg. 1994; 88 (suppl 1): 3-4.

49. White NJ, Walker D, Crawley J, Nosten F, Chapman O, Brewster O, Greenwood BM. Comparison of artemether and chloroquine for severe malaria in Gambian children. Lancet. 1992; 339: 317-321.

50. Kremsner PG, Luty AJF, Graninger W. Combination chemotherapy for *Plasmodium falciparum* malaria. Parasitol Today 1997; 13: 167-168.

51. Karbwang J, NaBangchang K, Thanavibul A, Ditta M, Harinasuta T. A comparative clinical trial of two different regimens of artemether plus mefloquine in multidrug resistant falciparum malaria. Trans R Soc Trop Med Hyg 1995; 89: 296-298

52. Martin SK, Oduola AMJ, Milhous WK. Reversal of chloroquine resistance in *Plasmodium falciparum* by verapamil Science. 1987; 235: 899-901.

53. Slater AFG. Chloroquine: mechanism of drug action and resistance in *Plasmodium falciparum*. Pharmacol Therap 1993; 57: 203-235.

54. Ginsburg H, Krugliak M. Quinoline-containing antimalarial - Mode of action, drug resistance and its reversal. Biochem Pharmacol 1992; 43: 63-70.

55. Krogstad DJ, Gluzman IY, Kyle DE, Oduola AMJ, Martin SK, Milhous WK, Schlesinger PH. Efflux of chloroquine from *Plasmodium falciparum*: Mechanism of chloroquine resistance. Science 1987; 238: 1283-1285.

56. Cox-Singh J, Singh B, Alias A, Abdullah MS. Assessment of the association between three pfmdr 1 point metations and chloroquine resistance *in vitro* of Malaysian *Plasmodium falciparum* isolates. Trans R Soc Trop Med Hyg 1995; 89: 436-437.

57. Basco LK, LeBras J. Reversal of chloroquine resistance with desipramine in isolates of *Plasmodium falciparum* from central and West Africa. Trans R Soc Trop Med Hyg 1990; 84: 479-481.

58. Basco LK, Ringwald P, LeBras J. Chloroquine-potentiating action of antihistaminics in *Plasmodium falciparum in vitro*. Ann Trop Med Parasitol 1991: 85: 223-228.

59. Peters W, Ekong R, Robinson BL, Warhurst DC. The chemotherapy of rodent malaria XLV. Reversal of chloroquine resistance in rodent and human Plasmodium by antihistaminic agents. Ann Trop Med Parasitol 1990; 84: 541-551.

60. Kyle DE, Oduola AMJ, Martin SK, Milhous WK. *Plasmodium falciparum*: modulation by calcium antagonists of resistance to chloroquine, *in vitro*. Trans R Soc Trop Med Hyg 1992; 84: 474-478.

61. Oduola AMJ, Omitowoju GO, Gerenah, Kyle DE, Milhous WK, Sowunmi A, Salako LA. Reversal of mefloquine resistance with penfluridol in isolates of *Plasmodium falciparum* from South-West Nigeria. Trans R Soc Trop Med Hyg 1993; 87: 81-83.

62. BitontiAJ SjoerdomaA *et al.* Reversal of chloroquine resistance in malaria parasite *Plasmodium falciparum* by Desipramine Science 1988; 242: 1301-1303.

63. Sowunmi A, Oduola AMJ, Ogundahunsi OAT, Falade CO, Gbotosho GO, Salako LA. Enhanced efficacy of chloroquine-chlorpheniramine combination in acute uncomplicated falciparum malaria in children. Trans R Soc Trop Med Hyg 1997; 91: 63-67.

64. Westman L, Kamanda S, Hellgren U, Ericson O, Rombo L. Rectal administration of chloroquine for treatment of children with malaria. Trans R Soc Trop Med Hyg 1994; 88: 446.

65. Salako LA WalkerO IyunAO. Pharmacokinetics of chloroquine in renal insufficiency. Afr. J Med Sci 1984; 13: 177-182.

66. Fu S, Bjorkman A, Wahlin B, Ofori-Adjei D, Ericsson O, Sjoqvist F. *In vitro* activity of chloroquine, the two enantiomers of chloroquine, desethylchloroquine and pyronaridine against *Plasmodium falciparum*. Br J Clin Pharmacol 1986; 22: 93-96

67. Abila B, IkuezeR Effects of Clemastine ketotifen and prednisolone on chloroquine pruritus in black Africans. Br J Clin Pharmacol 1989;27:116-117

68. Olatunde IA. Parenteral chloroquine in children. W Afr Med J 1970; 19:93-99

69. Williams ARF. Malaria in children. Br Med J. 1966; 2:1531-1537.

70. Riou B, Barriot P, Rimailho A, Baud FJ. Treatment of severe chloroquine poisoning. New Engl J Med 1988; 318:1-6.

71. Tanenbaum H, Tuffanelli DL. Antimalarial Agents. Arch Dermatol 1980; 116: 587-590.

72. Peets EA, Jackson M, Symchowicz E. Metabolism of chlorpheniramine maleate in man. J Pharmacol Expt Ther 1972; 180: 464-474.

73. Simons RFE, Luciut GH, Simons KJ. Pharmacokinetics and efficacy of chlorpheniramine in children. J Allergy Clin Immunol 1982; 69: 376-387.

74. Duke MNG In: Meyler's Side effects of drugs. Elsevier New York. 1992 12th edition Pp 366-372.

75. Ramsay AR, Msaki EP, Kennedy N, Ngowi FI, Gillespie SH. Evaluation of the safety and efficacy of micronized halofantrine in the treatment of semi-immune patients with acute, *Plasmodium falciparum* malaria. Ann Trop Med Parasitol 1996; 9: 461-466.

76. AkhtarT, Imran M.Sudden Deaths while on halofantrine treatment: A report of cases from Peshawar. J Pak Med Assoc 1994; 44:120-121.

77. Monlum E, LeMetayer P, Szwandt S, Neau D, Longy-Boursier M, Horton J, LeBras M. Cardiac complications of halofantrine :a prospective study of 20 patients. Trans R Soc Trop Med Hyg 1995; 89:430-433.

78. Warsame M, Werndorfer WH, Bjorkman A. Lack of effect of desipramine on the response to chloroquineof patients with chloroquine resistant falciparum malaria. Trans R Soc Trop Med Hyg 1992; 86: 235-236.

79. Boulter MK, Bray PG, Howells RE, Ward SA. The potential of desipramine to reverse chloroquine resistance in *Plasmodium falciparum* is reduced by its binding to plasma protein. Trans R Soc Trop Med Hyg 1993; 87:303-306.

80. Sowunmi A, Oduola AMJ, Ogundahunsi OAT, Salako LA.Comparative efficacy of chloquine plus chlorpheniramine and pyrimethamine-sulphadoxine in acute uncomplicated falciparum malaria in Nigerian children. Trans R Soc Trop Hyg 1998; 92 :77-81

81. Sowunmi A, Oduola, AMJ, Salako LA, Ogundahunsi OAT, Laoye OJ, Walker O. The relationship between the response of falciparun malaria to mefloquine in African children and its sensitivity *in vitro*. Trans R Soc of Tropical Med Hyg 1992; 86: 368-371.

82. Dean AG, Dean JA, Coulomber D, Brendel KA, Smith DC, Burton AH, Dicker RC, Sullivan K, Fagan RF, Arner TG. *Epi Info Version 6.A word processing database, and statistics program for public health on IBM-compartible microcomputer.* Atlanta, Georgia:Centers for Control and Prevention and Geneva: World Health Organisation 1994.

83. Bruce-Chwatt LJ. Malaria in African infants and children in Southern Nigeria. Ann Trop Med. 1952; 46: 173-178.

84. SowunmiA. Hepatomegaly in falciparum malaria in children. Trans R Soc Trop Med Hyg 1996; 90: 540-542.

85. Von Seidlein L, Jaffar S, Greenwood B. Prolongation of the QTc interval in African children treated for falciparum malaria. Am J Trop Med Hyg 1997; 50: 494-497.

86. Abdalla S, Weatherall DJ, Wickramasinghe SN, Hughes M. Anaemia of Plasmodium falciparum malaria. Br J Haem. 1980; 46: 171-183.

87. McGregor IA, Gilles HM, Walters JH, Davies AH, Pearson FA. Effects of heavy and repeated malaria infections on Gambian infants and children. Br Med J 1956; 2: 686-692.

88. Sowunmi A. Renal function in acute falciparum malaria. Arch. Dis Child 1996; 74:293-298.

89. Sowunmi A, Oduola AMJ, Ogundahunsi A, Fehintola FA, Salako LA. Pharmacokinetic interactions of chlorpheniramine and chloroquine in volunteers in Nigeria. Am. J. Trop. Med. Hyg (abstract) 1997.

Appendix 1

Calculation of sample size

Unmatched Cohort and Cross-Sectional Studies (Exposed and Nonexposed)
Sample Sizes for 50.00 % Disease in Unexposed Group

Conf.	Power	Disease Unex:Exp	Risk in Exposed	Odds Ratio	Ratio	Sample Size Unexp.	Exposed	Total
95.00 %	**90.00 %**	**1:1**	**90.00 %**	**1.80**	**9.00**	**30**	**30**	**60**
1.								
90.00 %	"	"				25	25	50
95.00 %	"	"				30	30	60
99.00 %	"	"				41	41	82
99.90 %	"	"				57	57	114
95.00 %	80.00 %	"				24	24	48
"	90.00 %	"				30	30	60
"	95.00 %	"				36	36	72
"	99.00 %	"				48	48	96
"	90.00 %	4:1				76	19	95
"	"	3:1				60	20	80
"	"	2:1				46	23	69
"	"	1:2				22	44	66
"	"	1:3				19	57	76
"	"	1:4				17	69	86

Formula : m' = Sq{c(a/2)*Sqrt[(r+1)*PQ]-c(1-b)*Sqrt[r*P1Q1+P2Q2]}
/(r*Sq[P2-P1])
m = .25m'*Sq{1+Sqrt[1+2*(r+1)/(m'r*Abs[P2-P1])]}

Reference : Fleiss, "Statistical Methods for Rates and Proportions",
2nd Ed., Wiley,1981, pp. 38-45.

GLOSSARY OF ABBREVIATIONS

ALP	alkaline phosphatase
ALT	alanine aminotransferase
AST	aspartate aminotransferase
CP	chlorpheniramine
CQ	chloroquine
Cr	creatinine
DNA	deoxyribonucleic acid
FBC	full blood count/ complete blood count
FCT	fever clearance time
G6PD	glucose 6 phosphate dehydrogenase
h	hour
HF	halofantrine
HR	heart rate
ht	height
KD	kilodalton
kg	kilogramme
min	minute
MPS	mefloquine/pyrimethamine/sulphadoxine
mm	millimeter
n	number
PCR	polymerase chain reaction
PCT	parasite clearance time

PCV	packed cell volume
Pd	parasite density
PR	pulse rate
RR	respiratory rate
SD	standard deviation
Temp	temperature
vs	versus
WBC	white cell count
x^2	chi square

The Dill-Glazko test

Add 50mg eosin powder to 100ml chloroform and 1ml HCl (1mol/1) in a glass-stoppered separating funnel. Shake gently for a 2 minutes until the chloroform becomes light yellow in colour. Separate the chloroform layer and store in a dry brown glass-stoppered bottle. Add 10 drops of the chloroform solution to 2ml urine in a test-tube and mix vigorously for about 2 minutes.

The presence of 4-aminoquinolines in the urine is indicated by a change in the colour of the precipitated chloroform layer from light yellow to violet-red.
Appendix 3

Lignin test

Place one or two drops of urine on a blank strip of newspaper or paper towel. Add a small drop of HCl (3mol/1) to the centre of the moistened area. The immediate appearance of a yellow to orange colour indicates the presence of sulphonamides and stays positive for 3 days.

Appendix 4

Giemsa stain

Thick films obtained by finger prick method are air dried for about 30 minutes. Slide is placed standing in the trays filled with giemsa stain for 15-30 minutes. Slide is rinsed in buffer water, and allowed to dry in air. To avoid precipitation of stains on the slides, the buffer must be precisely at pH 6.8-7.2.

Appendix 5

Microscopy

Microscopy was done using X1000 oil immersion lens and 6-7 eye piece. the dianosis of malaria was made by identification of the trophozoites in thick films stained with Giemsa. Quantification of parasites on thick blood films was done by counting the number of trophozoites against 1000 white blood cells and the amount per microlitre of blood derived according to following formula.

$$\frac{\text{Parasite counted}}{\text{Leukocytes counted}} \quad X \quad 6000 = \text{parasite count per microlitre}$$

The parasite count at day 0 was used as baseline and put at 100% for each patient. Further counts on subsequent days were expressed as a fraction of the count on day 0

Appendix:

Calculation of sample size[20]

Unmatched Cohort and Cross-Sectional Studies (Exposed and Nonexposed)
Sample Sizes for 50.00 % Disease in Unexposed Group

Conf.	Power	Unex:Exp	Disease in Exposed	Risk Ratio	Odds Ratio	Sample Size Unexp.	Exposed	Total
95.00 %	90.00 %	1:1	90.00 %	1.80	9.00	30	30	60
1.								
90.00 %	"	"				25	25	50
95.00 %	"	"				30	30	60
99.00 %	"	"				41	41	82
99.90 %	"	"				57	57	114
95.00 %	80.00 %	"				24	24	48
"	90.00 %	"				30	30	60
"	95.00 %	"				36	36	72
"	99.00 %	"				48	48	96
"	90.00 %	4:1				76	19	95
"	"	3:1				60	20	80
"	"	2:1				46	23	69
"	"	1:2				22	44	66
"	"	1:3				19	57	76
"	"	1:4				17	69	86

Formula   : m' = Sq{c(a/2)*Sqrt[(r+1)*PQ]-c(1-b)*Sqrt[r*P1Q1+P2Q2]}
                /(r*Sq[P2-P1])
          m = .25m'*Sq{1+Sqrt[1+2*(r+1)/(m'r*Abs[P2-P1])]}

Reference: Fleiss, "Statistical Methods for Rates and Proportions",
          2nd Ed., Wiley, 1981, pp. 38-45.

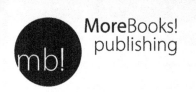

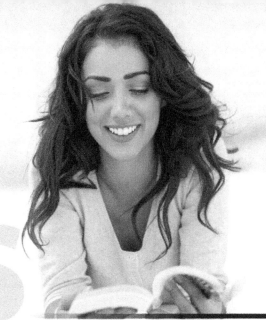

Made in the USA
Coppell, TX
18 March 2020